VARICOSE LEG ULCERS

THE ULTIMATE GUIDE TO DEALING WITH LEG ULCERS

DR. JUSTIN .TIMOTHY

Table of Contents

CHAPTER ONE 4
INTRODUCTION TO VARICOSE LEG ULCERS 4
    SIGNIFICANCE OF IDENTIFYING AND TREATING VARICOSE LEG ULCERS 9
CHAPTER TWO 15
    WHAT ARE VARICOSE VEINS? 15
    HOW DO VARICOSE VEINS CAUSE LEG ULCERS? 22
CHAPTER THREE 34
    SIGNS AND SYMPTOMS OF VARICOSE LEG ULCERS 34
    WHAT ARE YOU ABLE TO DO ABOUT VARICOSE LEG ULCERS? 38
CHAPTER FOUR 45
    WHO'S AT RISK FOR DEVELOPING VARICOSE LEG ULCERS? .. 45
    HOW CAN LIFESTYLE ALTERNATIVES REDUCE THE THREAT OF DEVELOPING VARICOSE LEG ULCERS? 53
    HOW VARICOSE LEG ULCERS ARE IDENTIFIED 58
CHAPTER FIVE 68
    WAY OF LIFE MODIFICATIONS THAT CAN ASSIST IN SAVING YOU FROM VARICOSE LEG ULCERS 68

SUGGESTIONS FOR ACCURATE CIRCULATION INSIDE THE LEGS 73

SIGNIFICANCE OF A NORMAL WORKOUT AND A WHOLESOME DIET 77

CONCLUSION OF VARICOSE LEG ULCERS 82

THE END 85

CHAPTER ONE

INTRODUCTION TO VARICOSE LEG ULCERS

Varicose leg ulcers are a commonplace circumstance that affects millions of human beings worldwide. It could be a source of soreness and ache for folks who suffer from it, and it can also lead to more extreme health headaches if left untreated. We will explore the reasons, signs, and remedy alternatives for varicose leg ulcers. Whether you have been recognized with this circumstance or are genuinely curious about studying more, Examine to gain a deeper knowledge of varicose leg ulcers and what you may do to manage them.

Varicose leg ulcers are a common health situation that impacts an enormous part of the populace. These painful and unpleasant sores can significantly impact someone's physical well-being and mental fitness. Information about the causes, symptoms, and treatments of varicose leg ulcers is crucial for anyone who wants to preserve their fitness and well-being. We can offer a complete introduction to varicose leg ulcers geared toward the majority. So, whether you are suffering from this situation or sincerely need to learn more about it, keep studying to learn all you need about varicose leg ulcers.

Varicose leg ulcers can be a painful and uncomfortable situation affecting many humans, particularly people with underlying vascular issues. They could greatly affect one's daily life, making it hard to move around and engage in normal activities. we can explore the topic of varicose leg ulcers in detail, looking at their reasons, signs, and treatment options. Whether or not you are currently dealing with this circumstance or inquisitive about mastering it, this will provide treasured insights that allow you to better apprehend and manage varicose leg ulcers.

Varicose leg ulcers are a common situation affecting hundreds of thousands of human beings worldwide. It can enormously affect someone's high-quality lifestyle and even cause extreme headaches if left untreated. We can outline varicose leg ulcers, their reasons, symptoms, and available remedy options. Whether or not you've been recognized in this situation or just curious to learn more about it, this post is for you. So, without further ado, let's dive in and explore the arena of varicose leg ulcers.

A varicose leg ulcer commonly affects thousands of humans worldwide, inflicting pain and ache. It is possible because of a spread of things, which include age, genetics, obesity, and way of life selections. Notwithstanding its incidence, many humans are unaware of this condition's signs and treatment alternatives. We can explore what a varicose leg ulcer is and how it affects the body. We can also discuss the diverse treatment alternatives, including lifestyle modifications, medicinal drugs, and surgical procedures. Whether or not you or a loved one are experiencing symptoms of a varicose leg ulcer or need to learn more about this circumstance.

Varicose leg ulcers can be a commonplace and painful situation affecting many people of all ages. They could cause pain, self-consciousness, or even incapacity if left untreated. But knowledge of the reasons, signs, and remedies for varicose leg ulcers can help individuals take control of their condition and improve their quality of life. In this article, we can introduce varicose leg ulcers and shed light on the important information everyone should realize.

SIGNIFICANCE OF IDENTIFYING AND TREATING VARICOSE LEG ULCERS

Varicose leg ulcers are a common problem affecting many of the populace. They are because of an expansion of factors, including terrible flow, weight problems, pregnancy, and genetics. Figuring out and treating varicose leg ulcers is crucial because they can result in various fitness issues if left untreated. We will discuss the importance of figuring out and treating varicose leg ulcers. Varicose leg ulcers are open sores that broaden the pores and skin due to terrible leg movement. They typically appear on the lower leg and can be painful, itchy, and uncomfortable. They can also cause swelling, redness, and discoloration of the skin. If left untreated, varicose leg ulcers can inflate, leading to more critical health troubles.

Figuring out varicose leg ulcers is important because they can indicate an extreme underlying circumstance. If you notice any of the signs stated above, it's critical to immediately consult your medical doctor. Your health practitioner will be capable of diagnosing the situation and suggesting the perfect remedy.

Treating varicose leg ulcers is essential because it can prevent the improvement of different fitness problems. The most common treatment for varicose leg ulcers is compression. Compression therapy entails sporting compression stockings or bandages to enhance flow within the legs. This could lessen swelling and help the ulcers heal more quickly.

In some cases, surgical treatment may be essential for varicose leg ulcers. A surgical procedure can help remove broken tissue and enhance circulation inside the affected location. This will help prevent other health troubles and enhance the overall quality of life for individuals with varicose leg ulcers.

In addition to conventional treatments, there are some domestic remedies for varicose leg ulcers. Those include preserving the affected region smooth and dry, elevating the affected leg, and warding off standing or sitting for lengthy durations of time.

Identifying and treating varicose leg ulcers is important for preserving fitness. If you notice any signs and symptoms of varicose leg ulcers, it's vital to seek your physician's advice immediately. Your doctor may be capable of diagnosing the situation and recommending the perfect remedy. Remember that early detection and treatment of varicose leg ulcers can assist in preventing the development of greater extreme fitness issues.

Varicose leg ulcers are a common yet painful circumstance that can develop in humans of all ages. These ulcers are often the result of untreated varicose veins, which can cause a range of headaches consisting of blood clots, leg swelling, and skin discoloration. Understanding the importance of figuring out and treating varicose leg ulcers is critical for preserving the most reliable fitness and quality of existence. One of the most significant reasons why identifying and treating varicose leg ulcers are vital is that these ulcers can cause significant discomfort and pain. The open sores can grow infected, leading to even more complications and discomfort. Moreover, varicose leg ulcers can indicate an underlying fitness problem, including vein disorders or diabetes, which can cause more severe fitness problems if left untreated.

It is also important to observe that varicose leg ulcers can considerably affect a person's daily existence, restricting mobility and inflicting emotional misery. They can also cause isolation and social withdrawal, making preserving a lively and pleasurable lifestyle tough.

Fortunately, numerous remedy options are available for varicose leg ulcers, including compression remedies, surgical treatment, and medicine. But early detection and treatment are vital for stopping similar headaches and promoting healing.

If you suspect that you could have varicose leg ulcers, it is crucial to seek clinical attention promptly. Your health practitioner can examine the severity of the condition and suggest the appropriate remedy alternatives. They may also recommend lifestyle changes, ordinary exercise and a healthy weight-reduction plan, to help prevent the condition from worsening.

Figuring out and treating varicose leg ulcers is important for maintaining good health and a satisfactory quality of life. If left untreated, those ulcers can cause tremendous pain and soreness, leading to greater health complications.

CHAPTER TWO

WHAT ARE VARICOSE VEINS?

Varicose veins are a not unusual fitness condition that impacts many human beings, particularly those older or with a family history of the circumstance. Varicose veins are enlarged and twisted veins frequently appearing as blue or crimson bulges on the legs. They occur when the veins inside the legs weaken or damage, causing blood to pool in the veins and making them more visible. The signs and symptoms of varicose veins can vary from man to woman. Some human beings can also revel in pain, swelling, or heaviness inside the legs, even though others might not have any symptoms. In some cases, varicose veins can cause extra-serious complications such as blood clots or ulcers.

So, what causes varicose veins? Numerous elements could contribute to the development of this condition. One of the most common is genetics. If your dad, mom, or grandparents had varicose veins, you'd also be more likely to have them. Different chance elements consist of weight problems, pregnancy, aging, and a sedentary lifestyle.

When you have varicose veins, numerous remedies alleviate your signs and symptoms and enhance the appearance of your legs. Compression stockings may be worn to help reduce swelling and enhance circulation, while lifestyle modifications that include exercise and weight reduction can also help improve symptoms.

For extra-severe instances, there are several clinical remedies to be had. Sclerotherapy entails injecting an answer into the veins to cause them to crumble and fade away. Endovenous laser therapy (EVLT) uses a laser to heat the vein and seal it shut, just as radiofrequency ablation (RFA) uses warmth to shut the vein. In a few cases, surgery may be necessary to dispose of the affected veins.

Varicose veins are an unusual and regularly uncomfortable condition that affects many humans. Even though several dangerous elements could contribute to their improvement, many remedy alternatives are available to help alleviate signs and enhance the appearance of your legs. If you are concerned about varicose veins, talk with your health practitioner or a vein specialist to decide the best route of movement for your character's desires.

Varicose veins are a common circumstance that impacts tens of millions of human beings worldwide. They are swollen, twisted veins seen just below the floor of the pores and skin and are most commonly observed inside the legs and feet. Varicose veins may be uncomfortable and ugly and can cause more severe fitness troubles if left untreated. In this article, we can discover what varicose veins are and what you can do to prevent and deal with them. Varicose veins arise when the valves within the veins are not working well. Commonly, those valves assist in preserving blood flowing in a single path towards the coronary heart. But while the valves grow susceptible or break, blood can waft backward and pool within the veins, causing them to swell and bulge. The veins end up enlarged and twisted and might appear blue or crimson.

Varicose veins can be due to various factors, including age, genetics, being pregnant, and being obese or overweight. Folks who spend long standing or sitting are also at increased risk of developing varicose veins. In addition to being unpleasant, varicose veins can cause aching, swelling, cramping within the legs, and a feeling of heaviness or fatigue.

Treatment for varicose veins depends on the severity of the condition. In some cases, lifestyle changes such as exercising regularly, maintaining a healthy weight, and avoiding long intervals of sitting or standing can help prevent varicose veins from worsening. Wearing compression stockings can also provide alleviation by improving flow and decreasing swelling. If these measures are insufficient, medical remedies, including sclerotherapy or laser therapy, may be advocated.

Sclerotherapy is a non-surgical operation that involves injecting a solution into the affected veins, causing them to shut and sooner or later disappear. Laser therapy uses heat power to destroy the veins, causing them to vanish over the years. Each treatment is minimally invasive and can be accomplished in a health practitioner's office.

For more extreme cases of varicose veins, surgical tactics consisting of vein stripping or endovenous laser treatment may be important. Those processes involve doing away with or sealing off the affected veins, permitting blood to float through wholesome veins.

If you are experiencing signs and symptoms of varicose veins, searching for scientific attention is crucial. While varicose veins won't be a critical health concern for anyone, they can lead to complications such as blood clots, skin ulcers, and continual venous insufficiency if left untreated. Your medical doctor will permit you to determine the best path of remedy for your specific situation.

Varicose veins are a common circumstance that can cause pain and embarrassment for many human beings. However, various treatment options exist, from lifestyle adjustments to minimally invasive tactics to surgery.

HOW DO VARICOSE VEINS CAUSE LEG ULCERS?

Are you laying low with varicose veins? They can be uncomfortable and ugly; however, did you realize they can also lead to a much more severe condition: leg ulcers? In this newsletter, we will explore how varicose veins can lead to leg ulcers and what you may do to save yourself from them. First, let's look at what varicose veins are and how they shape. Varicose veins are swollen, twisted ones that seem just beneath the skin's surface. They commonly arise in the legs and toes and result from weakened or broken valves inside the veins. Those valves commonly allow blood to drift upward from the legs and lower back to the coronary heart, but after they become weakened or broken, blood can pool inside the veins, causing them to extend and twist.

Varicose veins aren't generally harmful; however, they can be uncomfortable and lead to headaches such as leg ulcers. Leg ulcers are open sores that form on the skin of the legs and feet. They may be painful, take a long time to heal, and result in infection.

So, how do varicose veins result in leg ulcers? While blood pools inside the veins due to weakened or damaged valves, it may result in multiplied pressure inside the veins. This increased pressure can damage the tissues surrounding the veins, causing infection and, in the end, leading to the formation of leg ulcers.

Further to the extended strain, varicose veins can also cause changes in the legs and feet' pores and skin, making them more susceptible to injury and contamination. For instance, the skin may also end up dry and itchy, resulting in scratching and similar damage to the skin. Varicose veins can also cause discoloration and thickening of the pores and skin, making it harder for wounds to heal.

Stopping leg ulcers due to varicose veins starts with treating the underlying circumstances several remedy alternatives are available for varicose veins, including compression stockings, lifestyle changes, and, in some instances, surgery. Your physician can help you decide which treatment option is best for you based on the severity of your circumstances.

In addition to treating varicose veins, there are several steps you can take to prevent leg ulcers. Those encompass:

-maintaining your legs increased as much as possible.

Averting status or sitting for long intervals of time

Workout often to enhance flow

Maintaining a wholesome weight

-taking care of your skin by keeping it smooth and moisturized

In case you are experiencing varicose veins, it's crucial to talk to your medical doctor about treatment options to prevent leg ulcers from forming. With the right care, you can decrease the danger of headaches and keep your legs healthy and pain-free.

Varicose veins and leg ulcers are not unusual scientific conditions related to the lower limb. Many people will experience varicose veins at some unspecified time in the future of their lives, even as the occurrence of leg ulcers is particularly low. However, many human beings do not understand that varicose veins can cause leg ulcers if not handled correctly. Varicose veins are veins that have become swollen and twisted. They generally arise within the legs and feet, and they increase while the valves that help prevent blood from flowing back into the vein do not function properly. As a result, blood pools inside the veins, causing them to stretch and enlarge. Varicose veins may be due to various things, including genetics, pregnancy, weight problems, prolonged sitting, and aging.

While varicose veins do not cause aches or pains, they can result in various complications if left untreated. One of the most extreme headaches is leg ulceration. Leg ulcers are open sores that can broaden on the skin of the lower leg or foot. They can be painful, embarrassing, and tough to treat.

So, how do varicose veins lead to leg ulcers? Well, when blood pools within the veins of the legs, it may cause the skin to thicken and become discolored. Over time, this could cause irritation and damage to the tissues surrounding the veins. If the tissue damage is severe enough, it can cause an ulcer to form.

Moreover, the multiplied strain in the veins resulting from varicose veins can cause the pores and skin to become fragile and extra susceptible to harm. Even minor accidents and scratches or cuts can cause an ulcer, specifically if the wound is not well cleaned and dealt with. Ulcers, which can result from varicose veins, generally tend to shape at the interior of the ankle and are generally shallow and gradual healing.

The best way to prevent varicose veins from leading to leg ulcers is to treat the varicose veins as quickly as possible. This will involve a variety of treatments, including compression stockings, sclerotherapy; endovenous laser remedies, and surgical procedures. Depending on the severity of the varicose veins, one or more of these remedies may be vital.

If you already have a leg ulcer, it is essential to seek medical attention promptly. Your medical doctor will be able to determine the underlying cause of the ulcer and endorse the right treatment plan. Some treatment options for leg ulcers due to varicose veins include compression remedies, wound care, and surgical operations.

Varicose veins can cause leg ulcers if left untreated. When you have varicose veins, it's vital to look for clinical interest promptly to prevent headaches. If you have a leg ulcer, search for scientific interest immediately, as those can be severe and tough to deal with Patients can find relief from varicose veins and leg ulcers with proper care and interest.

Varicose veins are a commonplace situation that impacts almost one-fifth of the adult population in the U.S. It occurs when the veins inside the legs become swollen and twisted, inflicting unpleasant bulges and discomfort. Even though varicose veins may be a cosmetic difficulty for some people, they can also lead to more intense complications, such as leg ulcers. Leg ulcers are gradual-healing wounds that develop at the pores and skin of the lower leg, ankle, or foot. They generally arise because of poor circulation, which can arise while blood pools in the veins of the legs due to malfunctioning valves. As a result, the tissue within the affected location receives insufficient oxygen and nutrients, improving an ulcer.

In terms of varicose veins, a primary contributing issue is the accelerated strain on the veins, which results in fluid buildup within the leg's tissues. The strain exerted on the veins may be due to various factors, including status, sitting for long durations, pregnancy, weight problems, or a circle of relatives' records of the condition. Through the years, the accelerated pressure can cause the veins to weaken and stretch, leading to varicose veins.

As the circumstance progresses, the broken veins become much less effective at transporting blood again to the coronary heart, leading to blood pooling in the veins and, in addition, increasing the stress. This strain, in turn, results in irritation and, in the end, pores and skin breakdown, which could cause a leg ulcer.

Moreover, varicose veins can trigger an inflammatory response within the body, accumulating white blood cells in the surrounding tissue. This buildup of cells can cause additional harm to the encircling tissues and might contribute to developing a leg ulcer.

One of the fine approaches to preventing or manipulating leg ulcers due to varicose veins is to treat the underlying circumstances. This may involve lifestyle changes such as a normal workout, retaining a healthy weight, and avoiding extended intervals of standing or sitting. Compression stockings can also help alleviate signs of varicose veins by supporting the veins and enhancing blood flow to the legs.

In severe cases, more invasive remedies, including surgery or laser therapy, can be vital to remove or repair damaged veins. A healthcare company ought to be consulted to determine the best treatment route for people experiencing varicose veins and related conditions, including leg ulcers.

While varicose veins may seem minor, they can cause greater complications if left untreated. The improvement of leg ulcers in people with varicose veins is just one example of those complications. Taking steps to control or prevent the development of varicose veins can help enhance overall leg health and prevent extra-severe complications from developing.

CHAPTER THREE

SIGNS AND SYMPTOMS OF VARICOSE LEG ULCERS

Varicose leg ulcers are a common worry associated with untreated varicose veins. In truth, approximately 80% of all leg ulcers are caused by underlying venous sickness. Varicose leg ulcers can be painful and unsightly, and they might severely affect your first-class lifestyle. If you're experiencing any signs and symptoms of varicose leg ulcers, it's vital to try to find scientific interest as quickly as feasible. In this newsletter, we'll explore the most common signs and symptoms of varicose leg ulcers and what you can do to manipulate them. What are varicose leg ulcers?

Before we dive into the symptoms of varicose leg ulcers, it's vital to understand what they are. Varicose leg ulcers are open sores that develop on the pores and skin of the lower leg, commonly above the ankle. They're caused by persistent venous insufficiency, a condition wherein the veins in the legs cannot efficiently pump blood back to the coronary heart. This results in a buildup of pressure within the veins, which could cause them to bulge and become varicose.

Over time, the extended pressure inside the veins can cause the pores and skin to break down and form an ulcer. Varicose leg ulcers may be tough to treat and can take several months or years to heal completely.

The signs of varicose leg ulcers can vary depending on the severity of the circumstances. But there are a few common signs and symptoms you have to be aware of, which include:

1. Ache or soreness in the affected area: Varicose leg ulcers may be very painful, specifically when pressure is applied to the affected region. You can also revel in the aching or throbbing in your leg.

2. Swelling: Swelling within the lower leg is a common symptom of venous insufficiency. If you're experiencing swelling and other signs of varicose leg ulcers, seeking medical attention as quickly as possible is essential.

3. Discoloration: The skin around a varicose leg ulcer might also end up discolored, typically reddish-brown. That is

Before we dive into the symptoms of varicose leg ulcers, it's vital to understand what they are. Varicose leg ulcers are open sores that develop on the pores and skin of the lower leg, commonly above the ankle. They're caused by persistent venous insufficiency, a condition wherein the veins in the legs cannot efficiently pump blood back to the coronary heart. This results in a buildup of pressure within the veins, which could cause them to bulge and become varicose.

Over time, the extended pressure inside the veins can cause the pores and skin to break down and form an ulcer. Varicose leg ulcers may be tough to treat and can take several months or years to heal completely.

The signs of varicose leg ulcers can vary depending on the severity of the circumstances. But there are a few common signs and symptoms you have to be aware of, which include:

1. Ache or soreness in the affected area: Varicose leg ulcers may be very painful, specifically when pressure is applied to the affected region. You can also revel in the aching or throbbing in your leg.

2. Swelling: Swelling within the lower leg is a common symptom of venous insufficiency. If you're experiencing swelling and other signs of varicose leg ulcers, seeking medical attention as quickly as possible is essential.

3. Discoloration: The skin around a varicose leg ulcer might also end up discolored, typically reddish-brown. That is

because of the breakdown of purple blood cells while the skin is under stress for an extended period.

4. Itching or burning: Varicose leg ulcers may be very itchy or burn. That is because of the inflammation that occurs while the pores and skin are damaged.

5. Pores and skin modifications: The skin around a varicose leg ulcer can also thicken or harden. This is a signal of continual infection and can make the ulcer even more difficult to treat.

WHAT ARE YOU ABLE TO DO ABOUT VARICOSE LEG ULCERS?

If you're experiencing any of the symptoms of varicose leg ulcers, it's important to search for clinical interest as soon as possible. Your health practitioner can diagnose the condition and recommend a course of treatment.

Treatment for varicose leg ulcers normally involves addressing the underlying venous insufficiency. This may contain a compression remedy, which improves blood flow inside the legs and reduces swelling. Other remedies might include topical medicines, antibiotics to prevent infection, and surgical procedures in extreme cases.

Similarly to scientific treatment, there are numerous things you can do to control the signs and symptoms of varicose leg ulcers. These include:

1. Increase your legs: raising your legs above your heart can help reduce swelling and enhance blood flow. Attempt to increase your legs for at least a half-hour in numerous instances a day.

2. Hold a healthy weight: excess weight can strain your veins, making it more difficult for them to pump blood back to the heart. Keeping a healthy weight can help lessen your chance of developing varicose leg ulcers.

3. Exercise often: everyday exercise can help improve blood flow to your legs and reduce the danger of developing varicose veins. Strolling, swimming, and biking are all high-quality options.

4. Avoid sitting or standing for lengthy periods: prolonged durations of sitting or standing can place extra strain on your veins. Try to take breaks and flow around each half-hour.

Varicose leg ulcers can be a painful and unsightly consequence of untreated varicose veins. If you're experiencing any of the symptoms of varicose leg ulcers, seeking medical attention as quickly as possible is crucial. With the right treatment and lifestyle changes, you may manipulate the signs of varicose leg ulcers and enhance your lifestyle.

Varicose leg ulcers are a commonplace condition that affects many human beings around the world. They are due to persistent venous insufficiency, which results in blood pooling within the legs' veins. This blood pooling causes the veins to grow and become enlarged and twisted, improving varicose veins. If left untreated, varicose leg ulcers can cause a variety of signs that could impact your day-to-day existence. we can discuss the signs and symptoms of varicose leg ulcers and how you can control them. The first symptom of varicose leg ulcers is the appearance of a rash or discolored region on the skin of the legs. The pores and skin may become red, brown, or pink in shade and feel itchy or indignant. You can additionally notice that the skin feels thick or leathery, and it can cause small bumps or blisters.

Another common symptom of varicose leg ulcers is swelling in the legs and ankles. This swelling may worsen at the end of the day, making it tough to wear shoes or socks. In a few cases, the swelling can be so intense that it causes the skin to break down, improving open wounds or ulcers.

You could experience pain or discomfort in the affected location if you have varicose leg ulcers. This pain can be a dull ache or a sharp, stabbing ache, and it can be worse while standing or taking walks for long durations of time. The pain may be followed by a sense of heaviness in the legs in a few instances.

Ultimately, when you have varicose leg ulcers, you can observe that your legs feel tired, even after minimal activity. This will signal that your veins aren't functioning well and that your body must work harder to pump blood back to the heart.

If you are experiencing any of those signs, trying to find medical attention as quickly as possible is essential. Your doctor can perform a bodily examination and may endorse imaging assessments to assess the situation of your veins. Treatment alternatives may additionally consist of compression stockings, medications, or surgery, depending on the severity of your circumstances.

In addition to searching for scientific interest, there are several things that you could do at home to control the symptoms of varicose leg ulcers. These can also consist of elevating your legs whenever feasible, warding off lengthy periods of standing or sitting, and preserving a wholesome weight. You could also benefit from sporting compression stockings, enhancing circulation inside the legs and decreasing swelling.

Varicose leg ulcers can cause various signs and symptoms that could affect your daily life. If you are experiencing any of those signs and symptoms, trying to find medical attention as soon as feasible is critical. With the right remedy and self-care, you could manipulate the symptoms of varicose leg ulcers and enhance your quality of life.

CHAPTER FOUR

WHO'S AT RISK FOR DEVELOPING VARICOSE LEG ULCERS?

Varicose leg ulcers are a not uncommon worry of chronic venous insufficiency, a condition wherein the veins in the legs cannot efficiently pump blood again to the heart. As a result, blood pools in the veins, causing swelling, pain, and other uncomfortable symptoms. Even though all of us can develop varicose leg ulcers, certain elements can increase your risk. In this blog post, we will discover who is at risk for developing varicose leg ulcers and what you could do to prevent them. Age
Age is among the most important risk factors for developing varicose leg ulcers. As we age, the valves in our veins that help

to adjust blood flow weaken, making it more difficult for blood to flow back to the coronary heart. This may result in continual venous insufficiency and the development of varicose leg ulcers.

Gender

Ladies are more likely than men to develop varicose leg ulcers. This is partially because of hormonal modifications that occur during pregnancy, menopause, and other degrees of lifestyle. Hormones can weaken the partitions of the veins and cause chronic venous insufficiency, which increases the danger of developing varicose leg ulcers.

Family records

You'll be at extended risk when you have family records of varicose leg ulcers or other venous issues. Venous disorders can be hereditary, so if your mother, father, or siblings have had varicose leg ulcers, you will be much more likely to develop them.

Obesity

Being obese or overweight can increase your risk of developing varicose leg ulcers. Extra weight puts pressure on the veins in your legs, making it more difficult for blood to flow back to the heart. This could cause persistent venous insufficiency and the improvement of varicose leg ulcers.

Sedentary lifestyle

A sedentary way of life can also increase your risk of developing varicose leg ulcers. While you sit down or stand for lengthy durations of time, blood can pool within the veins of your legs, leading to swelling and different uncomfortable signs and symptoms. Every day workouts, which include taking walks or swimming, can enhance movement and decrease your chance of developing varicose leg ulcers.

Smoking

Smoking can also increase your chance of developing varicose leg ulcers. Nicotine and other chemicals in cigarettes can damage the walls of the veins, making it harder for blood to waft back to the coronary heart. This can lead to persistent venous insufficiency and the improvement of varicose leg ulcers.

At the same time that absolutely everyone can develop varicose leg ulcers, certain factors can increase their chances. Age, gender, circle of relatives histories, weight problems, a sedentary lifestyle, and smoking are all risk factors for developing varicose leg ulcers. In case you are in danger, there are steps you could take to lessen your risk, which include maintaining a healthy weight, exercising frequently, and quitting smoking. In case you are experiencing symptoms of varicose leg ulcers, which include swelling, aches, or pores and skin changes, it's important to seek clinical interest. Your physician will allow you to increase your treatment plan to manipulate your symptoms and prevent complications.

Varicose leg ulcers are a common yet debilitating circumstance that many people suffer from. It's essential to understand who's at risk for developing these ulcers so that the right prevention and remedy may be carried out. One of the primary risk factors for varicose leg ulcers is age. As we grow older, our veins become weaker and less elastic, which can lead to varicose veins and, ultimately, ulcers. Women are also more susceptible to developing varicose leg ulcers than men due to hormonal modifications that could have an effect on the strength and elasticity of their veins.

Weight problems are another threat to varicose leg ulcers. Excess weight places added strain on the veins within the legs, which could cause them to weaken and emerge as damaged. This may lead to the development of varicose veins and, finally, ulcers.

Those who have a family history of varicose veins or ulcers are also at increased risk. Genetics play a role in the improvement of those conditions, so if one or both of your parents have had varicose veins or ulcers, you may be more likely to have them as well.

Different hazard factors include a sedentary lifestyle, smoking, and certain medical situations, including diabetes and hypertension. Folks who spend long durations of time sitting or standing are at a higher risk for growing varicose veins and ulcers, as are folks who smoke. Excessive blood stress and diabetes can also weaken the veins and increase the risk of ulcers.

If you are at risk of developing varicose leg ulcers, there are steps you can take to prevent them from occurring. Maintaining a healthy weight, staying active, and sporting compression stockings can all help reduce the risk of varicose veins and ulcers. If you already have varicose veins, getting treatment for them can help prevent the development of ulcers.

There are numerous risk factors for varicose leg ulcers, including age, gender, and obesity, circle of relatives' records, a sedentary lifestyle, smoking, and positive medical conditions. By understanding these risk factors and taking steps to prevent and treat varicose veins, you can lessen the danger of growing ulcers and enhance your basic fitness and wellness.

HOW CAN LIFESTYLE ALTERNATIVES REDUCE THE THREAT OF DEVELOPING VARICOSE LEG ULCERS?

Varicose leg ulcers are a common condition that affects hundreds of thousands of human beings around the world. They're due to a selection of factors, but one of the most extensive is lifestyle choices. we will explore how lifestyle alternatives can reduce the hazard of developing varicose leg ulcers and what steps you may take to reduce your chance. First off, let's outline what varicose leg ulcers are. They may be open wounds that shape on the legs because of the negative stream. The situation results from weakened or broken veins inside the legs, which are not able to properly circulate blood returned to the heart, leading to blood pooling and infection. Varicose leg ulcers may be painful and unpleasant, and in intense cases, they can even lead to additional complications.

The best information is that there are steps you could take to reduce your risk of developing varicose leg ulcers. One of the best-sized elements that contributes to the situation is lifestyle. Here are some lifestyle choices that could increase your risk of developing varicose leg ulcers:

1. Sedentary way of life: A sedentary way of life can increase your chance of growing varicose leg ulcers. When we sit down or stand for extended periods, our blood flow slows down, which could cause blood pooling within the legs. This places a strain on the veins and might result in varicose

veins, which could sooner or later cause ulcers.

2. Weight problems: weight problems are any other lifestyle desire that could increase your risk of developing varicose leg ulcers. While we are overweight, we put extra stress on our veins, and this could cause them to weaken and become damaged over time.

3. Smoking: Smoking is a major hazard issue for varicose leg ulcers. Smoking damages the blood vessels and can result in a terrible stream, which exacerbates the circumstance.

4. Poor food plan: A terrible diet can also contribute to the improvement of varicose leg ulcers. A weight loss program high in saturated fats, salt, and sugar can lead to

irritation and a terrible stream that may worsen the situation.

Those are just a few way-of-life selections that can increase your danger of developing varicose leg ulcers. But there are steps you could take to reduce your danger:

1. Exercise frequently: everyday exercise can improve circulation inside the legs and reduce your risk of developing varicose leg ulcers. Attempt to incorporate a combination of aerobic exercise and energy schooling into your routine.

2. Preserve a healthy weight: preserving a healthy weight can reduce the stress on your veins and decrease your chance of developing varicose leg ulcers.

3. Give up smoking. Quitting smoking can enhance your overall fitness and reduce

your chance of developing varicose leg ulcers.

4. Consume a wholesome weight loss program: ingesting a wholesome food regimen that is rich in fruits, vegetables, and entire grains can lessen infection and improve flow, which may decrease your danger of developing varicose leg ulcers. Lifestyle alternatives play a giant role in the improvement of varicose leg ulcers. By making healthy lifestyle choices, such as exercising regularly, maintaining a healthy weight, quitting smoking, and eating a healthy diet, you could reduce the threat of developing this situation. If you are worried about varicose leg ulcers or any other health condition, be sure to speak with your physician for advice.

HOW VARICOSE LEG ULCERS ARE IDENTIFIED

Varicose leg ulcers are a common problem of chronic venous insufficiency, which takes place when the veins inside the legs are unable to successfully return blood to the heart. Those ulcers may be painful, unsightly, and hard to treat, but an early prognosis can cause better outcomes. So, how are varicose leg ulcers recognized? Here are some of the important methods that doctors may additionally use to pick out and compare this circumstance:

Physical examination:

Step one in diagnosing varicose leg ulcers is a radical bodily exam. Doctors will generally inspect the affected area, looking for signs and symptoms of pores and skin adjustments, consisting of discoloration, swelling, or hardening. They may additionally check for symptoms of contamination, such as a warm temperature, redness, and tenderness.

Scientific history:

Next, doctors will ask for approximately your clinical records, along with any underlying conditions that could be contributing to your signs and symptoms. This could encompass records of vein issues, diabetes, excessive blood pressure, or heart disease, in addition to any medicines or lifestyle elements that can be affecting your circulation.

Diagnostic exams:

To affirm a diagnosis of varicose leg ulcers, doctors may additionally use a ramification of diagnostic assessments consisting of:

1. Doppler Ultrasound: This noninvasive check makes use of sound waves to create pictures of the blood vessels on your legs, allowing doctors to assess the flow of blood and become aware of any blockages or abnormalities.
2. Ankle-Brachial Index (ABI) test: This simple test compares the blood pressure on your ankles to the blood pressure in your arms, allowing medical doctors to assess the severity of your venous insufficiency.
3. Blood exams: Blood assessments can help doctors become aware of underlying health conditions that may be contributing to your venous insufficiency, such as diabetes or anemia.
4. Wound subculture: If there are symptoms of infection, doctors may additionally take a sample of the wound to

determine the sort of bacteria or fungus that is inflicting the infection.

Remedy Plan:

Once a diagnosis of varicose leg ulcers has been made, doctors will work with you to develop a treatment plan that addresses your particular needs and goals. This can consist of:

1. Compression remedy: Compression stockings or bandages can help improve circulation and reduce swelling within the affected area.

2. Medicines: depending on the underlying purpose of your varicose leg ulcers, your medical doctor may additionally prescribe medications to help enhance circulation, lessen irritation, or treat infections.

3. Wound Care: The right wound care is important for healing varicose leg ulcers.

This may consist of ordinary cleaning and dressing changes as well as the use of topical ointments or dressings.

4. Lifestyle adjustments: Making lifestyle adjustments can also help improve venous insufficiency and decrease the risk of developing varicose leg ulcers. This will consist of losing weight, exercising regularly, avoiding prolonged intervals of standing or sitting, and sporting compression stockings.

Early prognosis and treatment of varicose leg ulcers are essential for stopping headaches and achieving the best feasible consequences. In case you are experiencing signs of venous insufficiency or have issues with varicose leg ulcers, make sure to speak with your doctor and discuss your remedy alternatives.

Strategies for treating varicose leg ulcers

Varicose leg ulcers are a common condition that impacts hundreds of thousands of humans worldwide. These ulcers may be painful and unsightly and can significantly affect a person's quality of life. Luckily, there are many techniques for treating varicose leg ulcers, ranging from easy home treatments to clinical interventions. We will discover some of the simplest treatments for this condition.

1. Compression therapy

Compression therapy is the most commonly used treatment for varicose leg ulcers. This remedy entails the use of compression bandages or stockings to enhance the flow of blood inside the affected location. The strain implemented by using the compression bandages allows for lessening the swelling and inflammation related to varicose ulcers and promotes recuperation.

Compression stockings and bandages are available in distinctive strengths, and your physician will prescribe the one that is suitable for your circumstances. Compression stockings should be worn at some point in the day and eliminated at night. They ought to be replaced every six months or as suggested by your health practitioner.

2. Wound Care

Wound care is another essential part of treating varicose leg ulcers. Right wound care consists of cleansing the ulcer, making use of a dressing, and keeping the affected region dry and smooth. Your health practitioner may additionally prescribe an ointment or cream to help heal the ulcer and save you from contamination. It is essential to comply with your medical doctor's instructions cautiously and to keep the affected area protected with a dressing to prevent further damage.

3. Surgical procedure

If compression remedies and wound care do not enhance the condition of your varicose ulcers, your health practitioner can also advocate a surgical operation. There are several surgical alternatives available, and your physician will propose the one that is satisfactory and acceptable for your condition. Surgical treatment can also include doing away with the broken vein, or it can involve repairing the valve inside the vein to prevent backflow of blood.

4. Laser remedy

Laser therapy is a minimally invasive technique that may help heal varicose ulcers. This procedure includes using a laser to wreck the damaged vein, which promotes restoration and improves blood flow in the affected area. Laser treatment is a secure and effective remedy choice for many sufferers with varicose ulcers.

5. Home treatments

In addition to clinical treatments, there are several home treatments that could enhance the circumstances of varicose leg ulcers. These remedies encompass:

elevating the affected leg to reduce swelling

applying a heat compress to the affected region to enhance blood flow

consuming lots of water to stay hydrated

Consuming a balanced diet rich in fiber and vitamins

Varicose leg ulcers may be a painful and debilitating circumstance; however, there are many effective treatments to be had. Compression therapy, wound care, surgical treatment, laser treatment, and domestic remedies can all help enhance the circumstances of varicose ulcers. If you suspect that you have varicose ulcers, it's vital to search for medical attention as soon as possible to save yourself similar damage and to get the treatment you want.

CHAPTER FIVE

WAY OF LIFE MODIFICATIONS THAT CAN ASSIST IN SAVING YOU FROM VARICOSE LEG ULCERS

Varicose leg ulcers are a painful and bothersome situation that affects many humans around the world. They occur when the veins in the legs emerge as damaged and cannot nicely convey blood back to the coronary heart. While this takes place, blood can pool in the veins, causing infection and regularly leading to the development of ulcers in the legs. While this situation may be hard to deal with, there are some lifestyle modifications that could help prevent varicose leg ulcers from growing in the first place.

1. Exercise frequently.

One of the best things you can do to prevent varicose leg ulcers is to work out frequently. Exercise enables your blood to flow properly through your veins, which can help prevent damage to the veins themselves. It can additionally help improve the muscle tissues in your legs, making it easier for them to pump blood back up to your heart.

2. Keep a wholesome weight.

Keeping a healthy weight is another crucial step in stopping varicose leg ulcers. Being obese places more stress on your veins, which can cause them to grow and break extra effortlessly. By maintaining a healthy weight, you may reduce the chance of developing varicose veins and related ulcers.

3. Raise your legs.

If you spend a lot of time sitting or standing, you may be in greater danger of developing varicose leg ulcers. To help prevent this, try elevating your legs as often as possible. This may help enhance blood float and decrease the amount of strain on your veins.

4. Put on compression stockings.

Compression stockings are a sort of hosiery that is designed to improve blood flow in the legs. They paint by applying strain to the legs, which allows the veins to push blood back up closer to the heart. In case you are at risk for varicose leg ulcers, your medical doctor may also recommend that you wear compression stockings to prevent them from developing.

5. Devour a wholesome food plan.

Eating a wholesome food regimen is another essential step in preventing varicose leg ulcers. A weight-reduction plan that is excessive in fiber and occasionally in saturated fat can help improve circulation and reduce irritation within the frame. This can reduce the chance of developing varicose veins and ulcers.

6. Avoid tight garb.

Sporting tight clothing, mainly around the waist and thighs, can place extra strain on your veins and increase the threat of developing varicose ulcers. To help save you this, try to wear loose, comfy clothing that lets in the correct movement.

Varicose leg ulcers may be a painful and irritating circumstance to address. But, by making a few easy lifestyle modifications, you may help prevent them from developing within the first region. By exercising often, preserving a healthy weight, elevating your legs, wearing compression stockings, ingesting a healthy weight loss plan, and avoiding tight clothing, you could help keep your veins healthy and reduce the danger of growing varicose leg ulcers. If you are at risk for this circumstance, speak with your health practitioner about other steps you could take to prevent it from developing.

SUGGESTIONS FOR ACCURATE CIRCULATION INSIDE THE LEGS

As we move about our daily lives, we often forget to attend to our legs. They carry us around, assist us in moving from one vicinity to another, and are frequently the most neglected elements of our body. One of the most essential factors in leg care is proper movement. The right move guarantees that our legs receive the important nutrients and oxygen they need to function well. we will make a few suggestions for selling excellent streams within the legs.

1. Work out regularly.

One of the great ways to promote excellent circulation inside the legs is to exercise often. A workout facilitates increased blood flow to the legs, which in turn complements the stream. Sports, which include walking, strolling, biking, and swimming, are all brilliant for enhancing movement within the legs.

2. Elevate your legs.

Another powerful way to promote top circulation is to elevate your legs. Raising your legs above heart level allows for less swelling and improves blood flow. While you're sitting or lying down, attempt to keep your legs improved with the use of a pillow or other supportive tool.

3. Wear compression stockings.

Compression stockings are designed to help improve circulation within the legs. They work by applying stress to the legs, which allows them to push blood back up closer to the coronary heart. Compression stockings are especially useful for people who are on their feet for lengthy periods of time, which include nurses, factory workers, and retail employees.

4. Avoid tight clothing.

Sporting tight clothing can restrict blood flow to the legs, which could lead to negative effects. Tight apparel can also increase the danger of growing varicose veins, which can be swollen and twisted veins that might be seen just under the pores and skin. To promote precise circulation within the legs, it's first-class to put on loose-fitting, comfortable clothing.

5. Preserve a healthy weight.

Being obese or overweight can put greater strain on the legs and decrease flow. Maintaining a wholesome weight via the right food plan and workout can help enhance movement and reduce the risk of growing leg-associated fitness troubles.

6. Stay hydrated.

Ingesting plenty of water is essential for good health. Dehydration can cause the blood to thicken, which could lead to negative effects. To promote accurate flow, it's essential to drink at least eight glasses of water per day.

Proper flow within the legs is crucial for normal leg health. By following these easy recommendations, you could improve circulation and decrease the risk of developing leg-associated fitness issues. Don't forget to exercise regularly, increase your legs, wear compression stockings, avoid tight apparel, keep a wholesome weight, and stay hydrated.

SIGNIFICANCE OF A NORMAL WORKOUT AND A WHOLESOME DIET

On the subject of living a wholesome lifestyle, there are two key additives that cannot be neglected: regular exercise and a healthy weight-reduction plan. At the same time, as it may appear to be a daunting assignment to incorporate both into your daily routine, the benefits of doing so are well worth the effort. We are able to speak about the significance of normal exercise and a wholesome food plan and how they work together to help you live an exceptional life. Normal workout Exercise is an essential part of a healthy way of life. It helps to keep your frame functioning efficaciously and reduces the chance of persistent illnesses consisting of diabetes, coronary heart disease, and a few styles of most cancers. There are numerous one-of-a-kind varieties of exercise that may be incorporated into your day-to-day routine, together with cardio, electricity training, and flexibility sporting events.

Cardiovascular exercise, including running or biking, helps improve the health of your coronary heart and lungs. This sort of exercise gets your coronary heart rate up and might help you burn calories and improve your metabolism. Strength training sporting events, which include weightlifting, can help to build lean muscle tissues that could enhance your average body composition. Finally, flexibility exercises consisting of yoga or stretching can help improve your variety of movement and decrease the risk of injury.

Not only does a regular workout increase your physical fitness, but it could actually have a superb effect on your mental fitness. Exercising releases endorphins, which are sense-top chemical substances that may help reduce stress and tension. Regular workouts can also help improve your sleep, which is important for universal health and well-being.

healthy weight loss program

The food we eat plays a big role in our universal fitness and well-being. A healthy diet can help prevent chronic diseases such as obesity, type 2 diabetes, and heart disease. A healthy eating regimen includes a variety of meals, inclusive of fruits, greens, entire grains, lean protein assets, and healthy fats.

Processed and packaged foods need to be limited, as they're frequently excessive in sugars, salt, and unhealthy fats. As a substitute, focus on eating whole, nutrient-dense meals that provide your body with the vitamins and minerals it desires to be at its best.

The significance of ordinary exercise and a healthy diet together

At the same time as ordinary exercise and a healthy diet are each critical additives to a healthy way of life, they're even more effective when used together. Every day workouts can help improve your digestion and metabolism, which could help optimize the blessings of a healthy weight-reduction plan. Exercise also helps to lessen inflammation throughout the body, which is mostly a result of a bad weight loss plan.

On the subject of weight reduction, everyday exercise and a healthy food regimen are vital. Exercise enables you to burn energy and improves your metabolism, just as a healthy food plan affords your body the vitamins it needs without adding extra calories.

A regular workout and a wholesome weight loss plan are two critical components of a healthy lifestyle. By incorporating everyday exercise into your daily routine and choosing nutrient-dense, whole ingredients, you could optimize your health and decrease your risk of chronic diseases. Don't forget small modifications can lead to huge outcomes, so begin by making small adjustments nowadays and see how they can positively impact your health and well-being.

CONCLUSION OF VARICOSE LEG ULCERS

Varicose leg ulcers are a common and persistent situation that could have an effect on each person. At the same time, as there's no permanent cure for the circumstance, there are various treatment alternatives to be had that may help control the symptoms and prevent the ulcer from recurring.

The primary reason for varicose leg ulcers is the damage to the veins in the legs, which results in terrible blood circulation. This may cause the improvement of ulcers in the lower legs. There are a variety of hazard factors that could contribute to the development of varicose leg ulcers, including obesity, pregnancy, and a family history of the condition.

One of the only remedies for varicose leg ulcers is compression therapy. Compression stockings or bandages are used to apply stress to the affected area, which helps improve blood flow and reduce swelling. This may help to hurry up the healing process and prevent the ulcer from worsening.

Another common remedy for varicose leg ulcers is the use of topical ointments or creams. These can help to lessen infection and promote healing of the affected area. In a few cases, antibiotics can also be prescribed to prevent infection.

Surgical options may be advocated in extra-severe cases of varicose leg ulcers. These can consist of approaches that include vein stripping or laser remedies to put off damaged veins and improve blood flow to the affected area.

In addition to clinical remedies, there are also lifestyle changes that can assist in the improvement of varicose leg ulcers. Those consist of maintaining a wholesome weight, staying energetic, and avoiding extended intervals of standing or sitting.

Varicose leg ulcers are a persistent condition that can cause discomfort and ache for those affected. While there's no permanent treatment for the condition, there are various treatments available that could help manipulate the signs and prevent the ulcer from recurring. In case you are experiencing any signs and symptoms of varicose leg ulcers, it's critical to discuss them with a clinical expert for an accurate analysis and remedy plan.

THE END

Milton Keynes UK
Ingram Content Group UK Ltd.
UKHW031833300124
436988UK00013B/858